Finding Motivation

For Your Fitness Routine

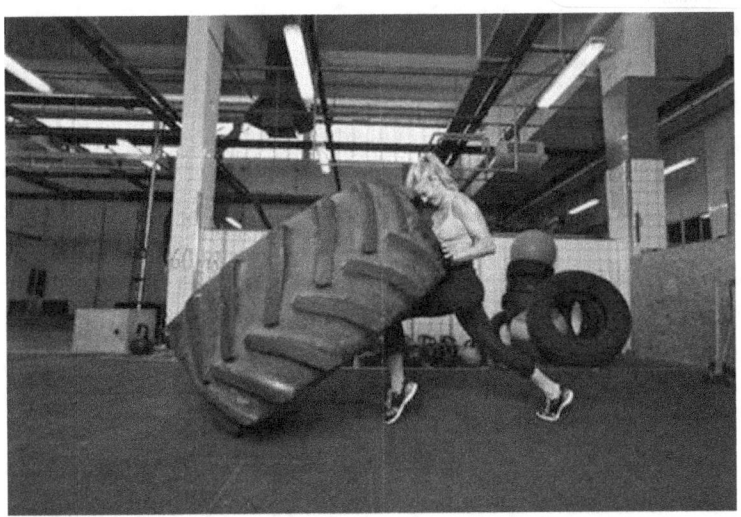

Health Learning Series

M. Usman

Mendon Cottage Books

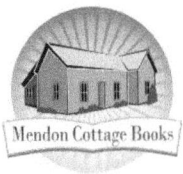

JD-Biz Publishing

Our books are available at

1. Amazon.com
2. Barnes and Noble
3. Itunes
4. Kobo
5. Smashwords
6. Google Play Books

Table of Contents

Preface

It is not easy to stick to a fitness routine. This is especially true when you are just getting started with exercising. Sometimes, you will not have the motivation to workout. Motivation is an important part of life. Without it, you would have no reason to work hard in life. Likewise, in its absence, you will have no energy to exercise.

Considering that physical activity is important, it is crucial to stay motivated all the time, so that you do not lose track of your fitness goals. Unfortunately, many believe that finding motivation is a difficult task. So, they start skipping workouts claiming they will hit the gym the day motivation will find them.

But, by waiting for motivation to find you, you only hurt your progress. Imagine what would happen if you went for a whole month without feeling motivated? Are you not going to put on weight during that time?

In this book, I will give motivation strategies to keep you exercising. Since we are all different, you will need to pick those strategies that will work for you. By the time you get to the end of this book, you will never complain of not having energy to workout.

Realizing your fitness goals will become a reality. If you have always wanted your watch to go a bit faster, your wish will come true. If you never had the energy to do extra sets, you will discover how easy it can be if you are motivated.

So without further ado, let's get started.

Introduction

Chapter # 1: The Reasons People Hate Exercising

It is a fact that people have embraced sedentary lifestyles. In the U.S. alone, 60% of the adult population does not engage in the recommended amount of physical activity. Of that, 25% does not get any physical activity at all. Considering the dangerous effects of an idle life, those percentages are shocking.

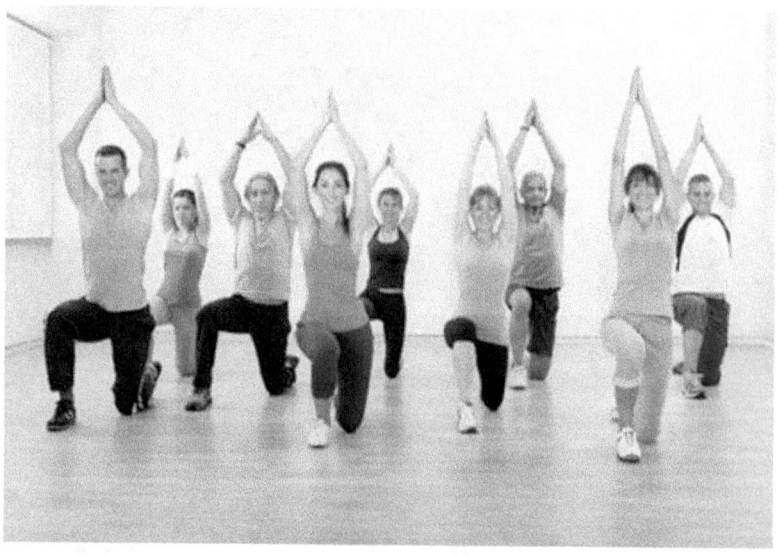

You might think that a human is not meant to be on his feet all day; dismissing an active life as something meant for wild animals. But, the truth is that humans are animals as well, and physical inactivity might be as bad as smoking.

The problem is that being lazy is enjoyable. You get to sit on the couch all day watching movies. If you spend most of your day at work, you probably have a nice chair in the office that's killing you. You view working out as something done by people with too much time on their hands.

Below are some of the reasons people do not have or lose the motivation to exercise:

Shooting for the stars from the start –

When you are a newbie in anything, it is not a good idea to hit maximum speed from the very start. Approaching your workouts with lots of momentum will leave you feeling exhausted. Then, before you will know it, you will have no energy to wake up for another exercise. The body needs to be given time to get used to any kind of vigorous activity.

Lack of knowledge –

Like everything in life, knowledge is important. You will need to know which exercises will give you the results you are looking for. At the same time, you must also know the right way of doing the workouts. In the absence of knowledge, you will find it difficult to reach your goals. Not only that, but you will also likely end up with an injury.

Not seeing results –

People exercise for a number of reasons, as some want to have a muscular body, some want to lose weight, and others just want to stay fit. However, often times, we think in extremes. We mistakenly see the transformation happening overnight, and, if it doesn't happen, we lose the motivation to exercise.

Too busy for a workout –

For many, this is the number one reason for not exercising. Taking care of the kids, education, work, and other activities fill the day, eliminating any chances of fitting in an exercise. Interestingly, the majority of those who are too busy to exercise still find time to sit on the couch and watch TV.

Exercising is boring –

There are others who just find exercising boring. However, there are a number of ways to make your workouts fun. For starters, you can try exercising with someone. Additionally, you can go for activities you enjoy, like swimming, gardening, hiking, etc.

Motivation is not something you have to wait for until it finds you. You have to take measures to find it, wherever it is hiding.

Chapter # 2: Benefits of Exercising

An active life is beneficial, regardless of who you are. But, for varied reasons, some of which were stated in the first chapter, many lose the motivation to exercise. However, if you want to live a full life, physical activity must be a normal part of your day. Here are some of the benefits of exercising:

Increased energy

Soon after a workout, you will feel a boost in energy. Exercising sends more blood and oxygen to your cells, giving you more energy. This is contrary to the misconception that exercising makes you feel tired and weak in the end.

Promotes good sleep

If you have trouble sleeping, chances are that you spend a good part of your day seated. If you start exercising, falling asleep will become easy. Additionally, you will notice that the quality of your sleep will improve, and you will wake up energetic, resulting in productivity throughout the day. Just avoid exercising too late, as that will leave you with a lot of energy, reducing your chances of going to sleep.

Controls weight

If you eat constantly and then spend the rest of the day on your couch, you must prepare for the worst. Regular physical activity ensures that you will maintain a healthy weight, which helps in the prevention of obesity-related diseases.

Increases confidence

When you engage in workouts, you start feeling good about your body.

Losing fat, gaining muscle, etc., are all activities that will make you proud of your body. This increased confidence will translate into other aspects of your life.

Improves mood

Working out releases hormones, which play a major role in determining your mood. If you had a bad day at the office, exercising is a better remedy than resorting to beer or smoking.

Motivational Strategies

Chapter # 3: Exercise with a Friend

Exercising with someone you like can be a game changer. As the old saying goes, "There is strength in numbers". Exercises that are boring and challenging can become easy and fun with the right friend. And, if you are feeling down on some days, your friend will give you the extra push, knowing you will return the favor someday. Let's look at the benefits of working out with a friend:

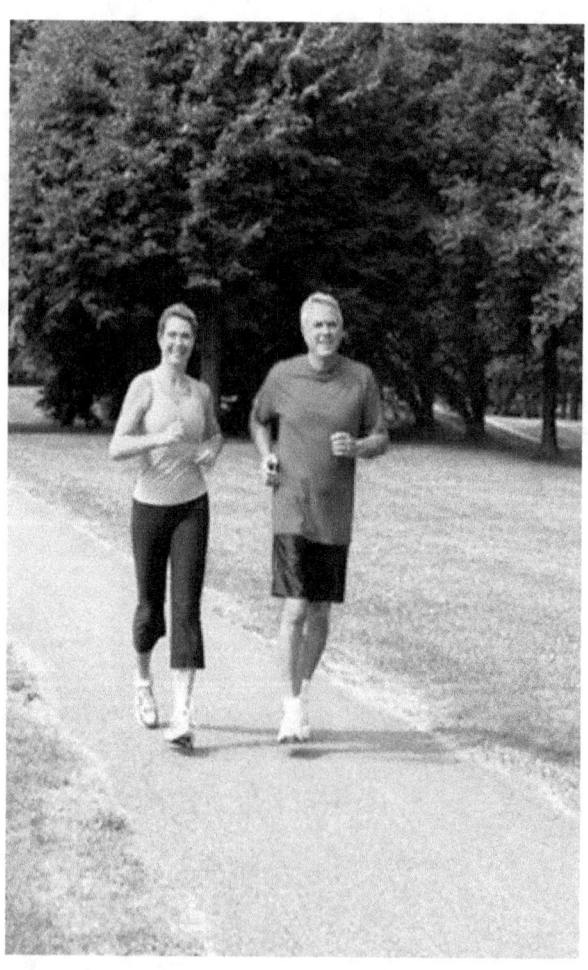

You will do more

When exercising with your friend, you will be motivated to do as much as they are doing. Even when you are feeling tired, you will push yourself to go on. In the end, you will find that achieving your dream is not as hard as you previously thought.

1. You will do the exercise longer

Since you will be chatting during the exercise, you will realize that finishing what feels like hours when alone, only takes minutes when with your buddy. This is especially true with exercises like walking and jogging.

2. You will feel accountable

If you fail to show up for the workout, you will have questions to answer. If your excuses are not valid, your buddy will help you overcome your weaknesses.

3. You will never miss a workout

You probably do not miss a date with your best friend often. When you have a workout buddy you love to hang out with, the chances of missing a workout will be very low. Although you might not love the actual exercise, you will always be looking forward to meeting your friend. With time, exercising will become a habit.

How to Choose a Workout Buddy

Not every friend will give you all the benefits you are seeking. With the wrong choice, you will realize that making a mistake is worse than having no workout buddy in the first place. So, here are some important things you must consider:

Same level of fitness –

It is a good idea to ensure that you share the same fitness level with your partner. If not, keep searching for somebody else.

Similar interests -

If you are trying to lose weight, go for someone with the same goal. Otherwise, you will want to run when he wants to bench press.

Someone you like –

Since you will be spending your time with this person, sweating and bleeding together, you must make sure that he is someone you like.

Chapter # 4: Be Prepared

The saying "Failing to prepare is preparing to fail" sums up one fact of life perfectly. Many do not feel motivated to workout simply because they did not take time to prepare. The mere thought of exercising starts a battle in the head.

One part will want to get up and sweet, because it knows the benefits of such an activity. On the other hand, another part will want to sit and relax. It is usually this second part that mostly wins. However, you can reduce the chances of that happening with just one trick. Preparation!

That begins with having your workout gear in place. For example, if you go for a run in the morning, it is not easy to get up and go into another room just to search for your workout clothes. But, if you put them on the floor when going to bed, it becomes easier.

If you use music, it's also a good idea to have your playlist ready before the workout. Adding to that, you must also consider having an exercise schedule. With this, you will know when it is time to sweat. So, if you were busy with something, fitting in your workout will not be so difficult.

Likewise, if your friends know your workout timetable, the risk of being disturbed by them will be very low. And, since you must change your workouts every time, you will also discover that it pays to know which exercise you will do beforehand. Trying to decide whether you should run or do strength training when the time is due is a guaranteed way to give your second side the power to take over.

Chapter # 5: Work with a Coach

You might not feel motivated to workout if you are not sure of what to do. It is important to know the types of exercises that are most effective, and also the proper way of doing them. Otherwise, you will find it helpful to work out with a coach.

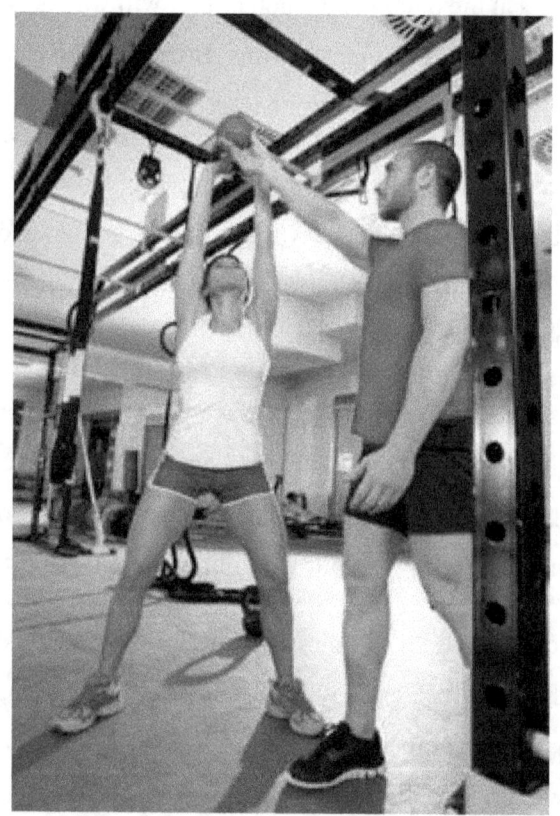

Everyone is different. If you are not seeing results with exercises that worked on someone else, you might start to feel unmotivated. However, this is simply normal. It is probably that there is something you are not doing right. But, when you have a trainer, he will give you advice and correct your mistakes. At the same time, he will give you additional tips for success.

And since coaches cost money, it is a motivator, as you will want to get your money's worth. If you do not show up that day, you will be the loser.

However, you should be careful when choosing a coach. Saying he is qualified is not enough to make him a good choice. Look at his experience, the people he has worked with, and anything you deem necessary. If you are convinced that he is the best option, then you can go ahead and work with him.

Chapter # 6: Take Part in Competitions

It feels good to be called a champion. Being successful against your competitors makes you proud. The good thing is that competitions are everywhere in everyday life. They include football, netball, swimming, wrestling, etc. You will likely find some of these competitions in your area. If you know you can make it, you are encouraged to join.

Taking part in such activities works for you in two ways: firstly, you will have a chance to win prizes. Secondly, you will be motivated to stay active every day, so that you are successful when the time to perform comes.

So, if you are trying to lose weight, you will easily achieve that without even thinking about it. If you wanted to get muscular, you can join a weightlifting competition, and, at the end, you will likely gain more muscle than you imagined.

In case you do not find any events that are in line with your goals, then you can take the lead and host a competition you want. You only need to find people with similar interests. For example, you can have a group of people who want to lose weight. You would say, "Whoever loses more weight by a given date will be the winner."

If you are looking for something fun, you can have regular dancing competitions. Since dancing is also an activity that burns fat, you will discover that you have lost weight in the end.

Having a competition it does not mean you should involve a lot of people. As a matter of fact, two people can have a great competition. If you do not get along with others well, you can even compete with your previous scores.

Chapter # 7: Reading Fitness Material

When losing weight, gaining muscle, or trying to achieve any fitness goal, it may feel like you are alone. You may even think that you are being delusional and that what you are dreaming of is not realistic. But, if you have someone showing you constantly that it can be done, you can use that as motivation and continuously work on achieving your goal.

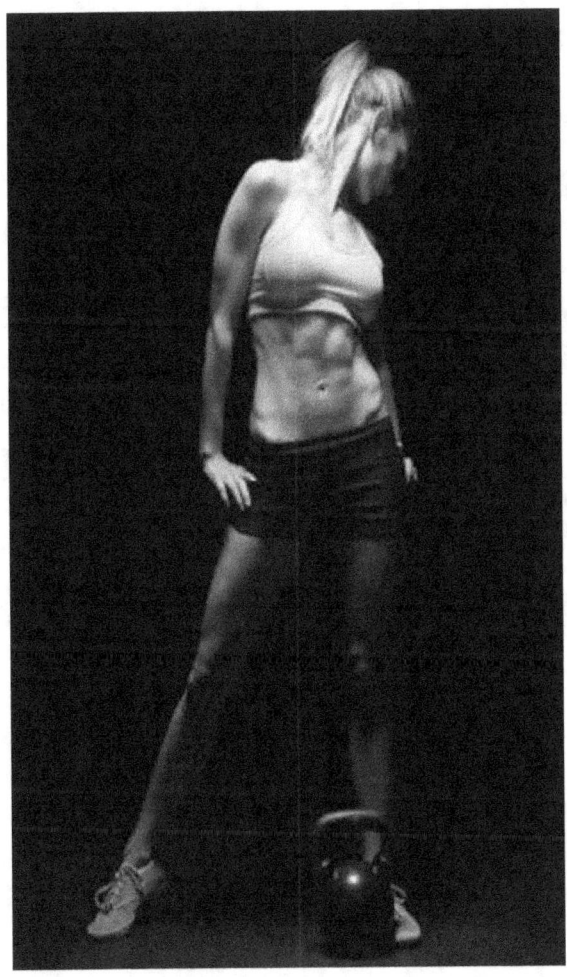

Mostly, it's magazines and blogs that carry motivational fitness content. However, you will also get this kind of information in other mediums. You will find success stories, tips on how to overcome your challenges, and more.

By just reading this kind of material from time to time, you will be inspired to go out and work. With time, you will get used to exercising and you will no longer need a magazine or a blog to motivate you.

Where to Start

Your local market is probably filled with a number of fitness magazines. Browse these and choose the ones you like. If you do not find good ones locally, you can turn to the internet where you will have a huge range of options.

Those who are not into magazines can turn to blogs. Again, there are so many of these on the internet, that finding one that will fulfill your needs will not be that difficult. The other reason I love blogs is that they can be accessed almost anywhere. You will be able to read them on your phone, in bed, and other places where a magazine will not be ideal. Making blogs even better, there is no need to pay for their content most of the time.

Chapter # 8: Join a Forum

While reading fitness blogs, magazines, etc., can be effective in motivating you, sometimes it is hard to believe the content in these mediums. You always have a feeling that some of the before and after photos have been Photoshopped. It's also normal to think that the guy claiming to have lost 20 pounds has been paid to write his success story and that he was not overweight in the first place.

This is where forums come to the rescue. However, do not be fooled into thinking that every member of a forum is there with good intentions; fraudsters are also present. But mostly, forums consist of ordinary Joes wanting to meet like-minded people.

If there is something that's bothering you, a forum is a great place to seek help and get motivated to keep exercising. While you will not get expert answers, hearing an honest opinion is better than a marketing pitch.

Furthermore, you will build relationships with real people. The best part is that these are people struggling with troubles similar to yours. If there is something you have been ashamed of, a forum is the best place to share it with people who can relate.

Although it is not mandatory to contribute to every conversation, it pays to be an active member. Besides, it's participation that makes forums grow and become a resource for everyone interested in its topics.

Another thing I like about forums is that there is no payment required. As long as you fit a certain criterion, you will be allowed to become a member.

Since there are so many of these on the internet, I would recommend that you do your research and join the ones you think will be suitable for you.

Chapter # 9: Log Your Workouts

Sometimes, it's the little things that make a big impact. If you are struggling to stay motivated with your workouts, perhaps a simple notebook might be just what you need to keep going.

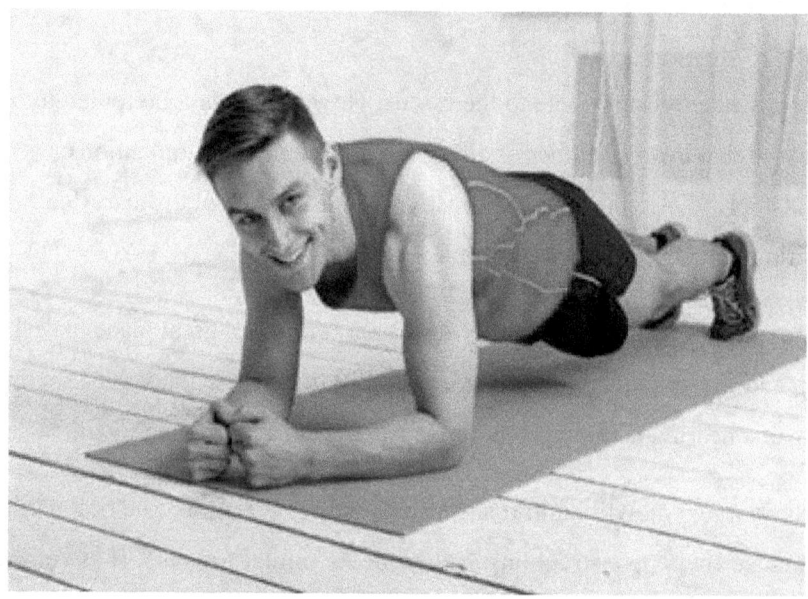

We constantly lie to ourselves that our brains are capable of remembering everything. But, the fact is that we cannot see everything from memory clearly. We only recall the biggest moments and neglect everything else. However, it is the little things in life that usually count.

Here is how logging your exercises will help you:

It will act as a reminder –

Logging your exercises will act as a reminder of the little achievements you made while you were working out. It could be that you managed to run a distance of one mile, which is something you were not able to do before.

You will notice improvement –

If you were sweating with 8 reps before, finishing 12 reps without feeling exhausted might not seem like much. And if you only keep this in your head, you will likely treat it as one of those things. But if you have a journal, you will notice easily that you are making progress and you will strive to keep the pace.

It will show you direction –

Keeping everything in your head might blur your vision, considering that you have a lot of deal with. But if you log your workouts, you will easily see where you are coming from and where you plan to go.

Where do you start

If you have not been logging your workouts, all is not lost. Starting today, have a notebook. Every day after a workout, record how much you did, the type of exercises, and anything else you deem necessary.

You can even use an application instead of a notebook. Since there are a lot of applications to help you in keeping track of your exercises, you will need to spend some time researching.

Chapter # 10: Rewarding Yourself

One way to stay motivated is by giving yourself a reward every time you achieve a goal. If there is something you have always wanted to own, you can set that as a reward you will get upon reaching your fitness dream. This will ensure that you do not quit exercising.

I have discovered that the reward is more inspiring if it is a luxury good. For example, if you love 3D games, you can treat yourself with a virtual reality headset. The reason basic needs do not work for me is that I will still go and buy them, even if I do not achieve the goal.

However, tastes differ. Others may be motivated with a basic need. So, whatever you know will work for you, go with it.

How to reward yourself

Firstly, you will need to determine a goal, e.g. lose a certain amount of weight. The next step is to set aside a certain amount of money that will be enough to buy the reward you want. Make sure that your goal is measurable and time-specific, as that will make it easy for you to know if you have achieved it or not.

When you have successfully fulfilled the goal, reward yourself. If you haven't been successful, do not cheat simply because you have the money. Instead, give it to someone you do not like or use it towards a cause you do not believe in. By doing that, you will be angry with yourself for failing to fulfill the goal. Then, the next time you try, you will likely give it enough effort, increasing your chances of success.

Chapter # 11: Sign a Contract

While the idea of signing a contract when you are trying to get fit may seem absurd, the truth is that it helps. There is no one on earth who likes to be called a failure. So, if the whole world knows that you want to achieve a certain goal, you will work at it in fear of embarrassment.

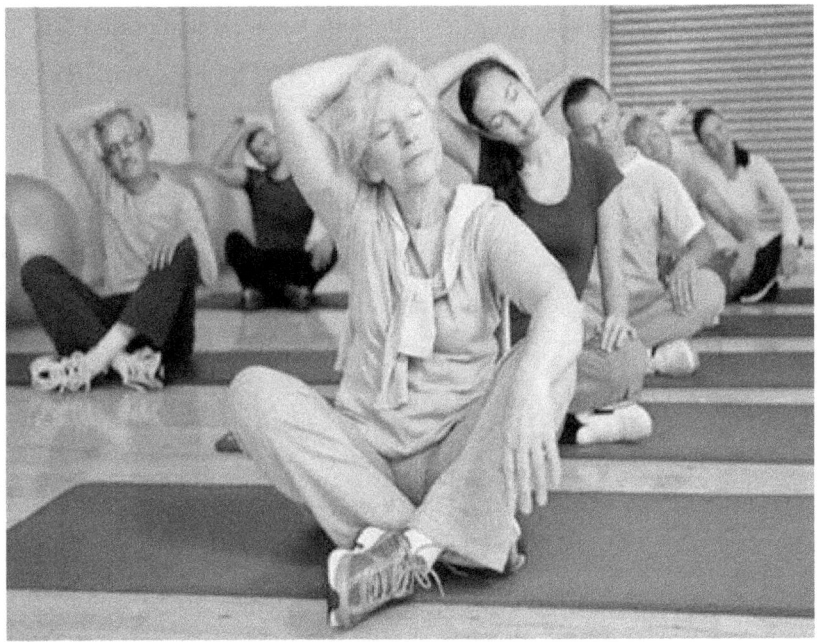

The contract does not need to be complicated or similar to the one you get when starting a new job. It just needs to show the goal you are trying to achieve and the time you expect to achieve it.

How to do it

Firstly, you will need to have a clear goal with a given time frame. Once that is in place, reach out to your friends and family to act as witnesses. Without other people involved, you will not be motivated to keep working out.

Your contract can be in written form or you can just agree through word of mouth. But you should preferably have it on paper.

The contract must also show what the consequences of not achieving the goal will be. For example, you can set aside an agreed amount of money that you will have to pay if you fail to be successful. If money is not an option, you can agree to not watch your favorite show for a defined period. Whatever you know will work as a punishment will be a good motivator. The stiffer the punishment, the harder you will exercise to achieve the goal.

Finally, you must also agree on how you will monitor progress. For example, if losing weight, you may get on a scale every week to determine how good you are doing. Just make sure all your witnesses are involved in the process.

Chapter # 12: Use Music

Music is one thing we cannot do without. Every time anyone wants to have fun, music is usually one of the recipes on the menu. It is used in weddings, parties, etc. However, what you might not know is that listening to your favorite music can also do wonders in regards to your workout.

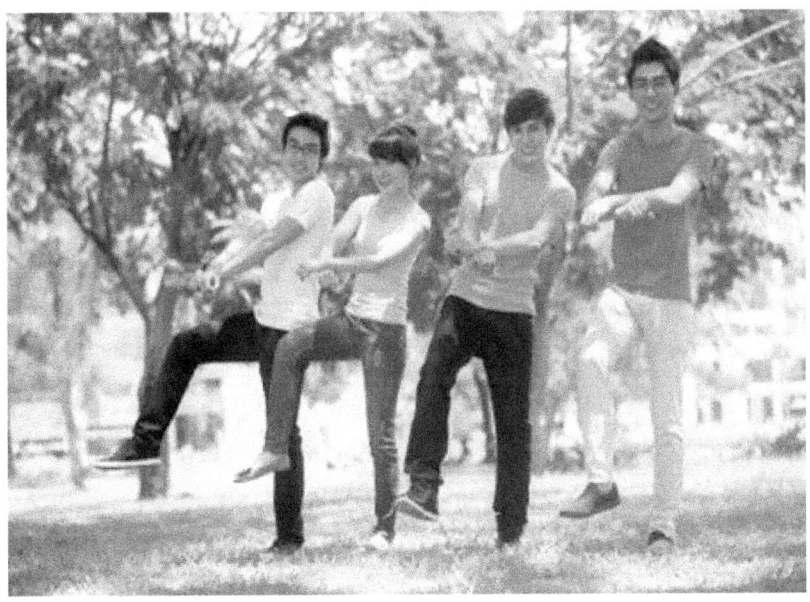

In a study where participants listened to music while exercising, it was discovered that their performance increased. Music is known to distract you from the pain and fatigue that is associated with exercising. Your body will focus on listening and moving to the beat. Although you might not find the exercise easier, you will have the energy to go on until you reach the finish line.

If you are one of those who find exercising as boring, music can make it fun.

Once you turn the volume up and select your favorite tracks, it will not be too long before your watch will be reminding you that you have exceeded your training time.

How to make a playlist

Although music will help you stay motivated to work out, it is not all music that achieves that, it's only fast-paced music that works. Specifically, your workout playlist should consist of music with beats per minute (BPM) of 120–140.

If it is slower than that, the music will not achieve the intended purpose. But, you must remember that different exercises will require different tastes of music. For example, if you are doing strength training, hip-hop will be the best option. However, that kind of music usually has lower BPMs.

I would recommend that you try different genres of music. As the old saying goes, "Variety is the spice of life." Changing your music every time will guarantee that you do not get bored with the same songs. However, remember one thing - nothing beats a BPM of 120–140.

Chapter # 13: Setting Goals

When you get into an exercise program, it's important to set goals. Not knowing what you are trying to achieve is a recipe for disaster. You will find no reason to wake up early to exercise. You will opt to stay in bed when it is cold. You will want to watch TV when you get home, claiming you are tired from work. All that sums up to one thing: not having goals will kill your motivation for exercising.

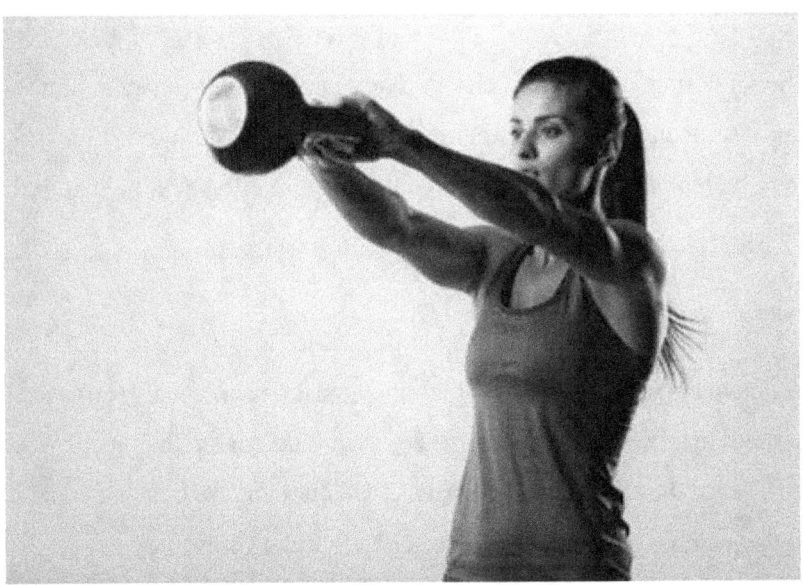

How do you set goals

The process of setting goals in not that complicated. What you first need to do is have the goal clearly determined. Are you trying to build some muscle? Are you trying to lose weight? Or do you want to just keep fit? It is important to work on a single cause at a time.

Having done that, you will need to ensure that your goal fits a certain criterion.

Measurable:

If your goal has no way to be measured, then you are as good as not having a goal in the first place. For example, if you are trying to lose weight, you will know if you are making progress by getting on a scale every week. Positive results will keep you motivated, ensuring that you will keep working out.

Achievable:

At the same time, you should ensure that your goal is achievable. Simply because someone did it does not mean you can easily do it too. You will need to be realistic. The bigger the goal, the more effort will be required to be successful.

Timely:

Goals must be given a time by which they must be achieved. However, remember that people are different. So, as you determine the time it will take to get to the finish line, be realistic. Do enough research and come up with the average time you expect to see the results you want.

I have found that if you have a bigger goal, it can be intimidating and result in demotivation. But, if you set smaller goals, like losing 2 pounds every week, you will find that you are motivated to meet the smaller goals. Before you will know it, you will have reached your overall goal, which might be to lose 20 pounds.

Chapter # 14: Visualize the Benefits

Constantly thinking about the benefits of exercising is one of the most effective ways to stay motivated. This technique has been used for years proving that it does work. In this chapter, I will show you how you can make use of it.

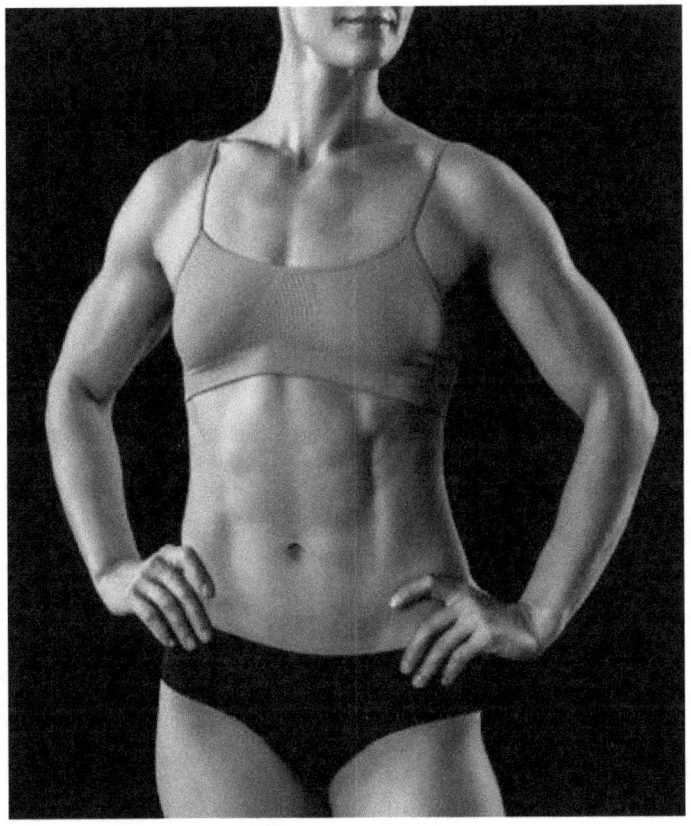

How it works

Being successful in achieving your fitness goals needs more than just your physical ability. You may be the strongest person on earth, but if your mind is not willing to excel, you will have a difficult time reaching your goals. Most of the time, when one quits exercising, it is because the brain is not providing the fuel to get him moving.

Although it is not easy to control the brain, you can still influence its actions. The truth is that the brain does what it wants. But with visualization, you can trick it to start pushing you into exercising.

For example, if you go out and exercise, you will have a great body. Clothes will start looking good on you. Your image will improve and so will your confidence.

Likewise, you can visualize that by exercising, you will become athletic. Your body will be responsive and you can imagine yourself doing some really cool tricks. By doing this, your brain will starting pushing you to workout.

When the time for action comes, you will find it easier to dig deeper for one more set. Going the extra mile will feel rewarding, as you know you will lose weight and prevent obesity-related diseases.

How to do it

Learning to visualize the benefits you will get from an exercise is not difficult. Start by taking a piece of paper. As stated previously, it is important to have a clear goal, which will make it easy to come up with the benefits.

Write a list of all the benefits that relate to the type of workouts you will be doing. Read each one of these benefits aloud. See how perfect your life will become once the benefit has transformed you. Let your mind ponder on each benefit and enjoy it, as if what you are visualizing is really happening.

For better results, you will need to keep visualizing all the time. The more you do it, the better. I would also recommend that you practice this technique just before and during the exercise.

Conclusion

It is not easy to feel driven for an exercise every time. On some days, you will not have the motivation to get on the treadmill or hit the gym. But with time, exercising will become a habit. You will not see it differently from brushing your teeth in the morning. When it gets to this, you will reduce your reliance on motivation when you want to workout.

Your body needs time to get used to physical activity if you have been a couch potato. So, do not be hard on yourself. Start slowly and increase the intensity as you go.

You should never waste time waiting for motivation to knock on your door. It is always inside you. All you need to do is figure out ways of bringing it out. Use the motivational strategies in this book. I would recommend that you start with those strategies you know will give you the best results. But at the same time, do not neglect the others. Remember, variety is the spice of life.

Exercising is important for everyone. Not only does it make you fit, but you also control your weight, boost your immunity, improve your looks, and more.

Regardless of who you are or what you do, physical activity must be a normal part of your day. Furthermore, you should also limit the time you spend sitting. If you follow those tips, you will certainly live a healthy and long life.

Thank you for reading and best wishes!

Author Bio

Muhammad Usman is a distinguished medical graduate of Allama Iqbal medical college (AIMC). He is a professional writer who has been in the field for more than 4 years. During this time he has produced 10,000+ articles, blogs, and eBooks on various niches related to diseases, health, fitness, nutrition, and well-being. He is a regular contributor to several journals related to medicine and surgery. He is the editor of several journals and newspapers.

Check out some of the other JD-Biz Publishing books

Gardening Series on Amazon

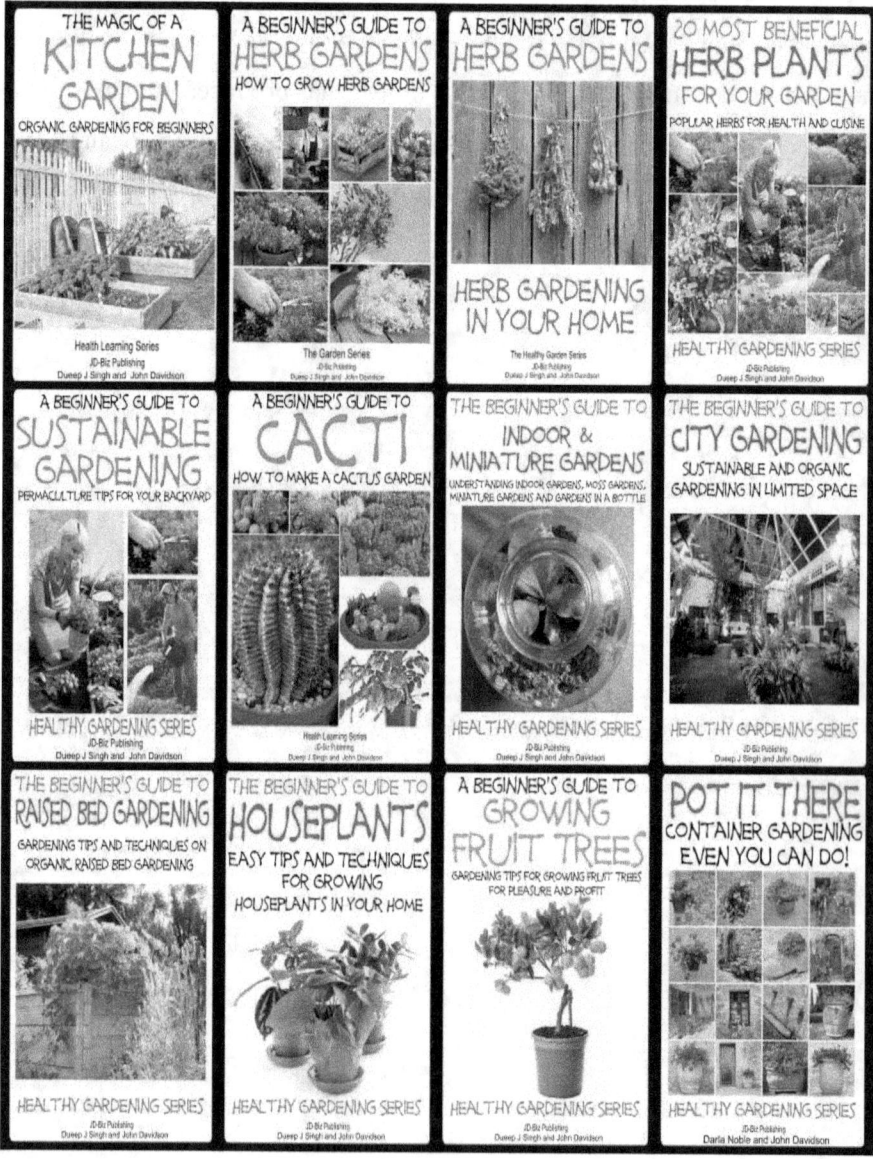

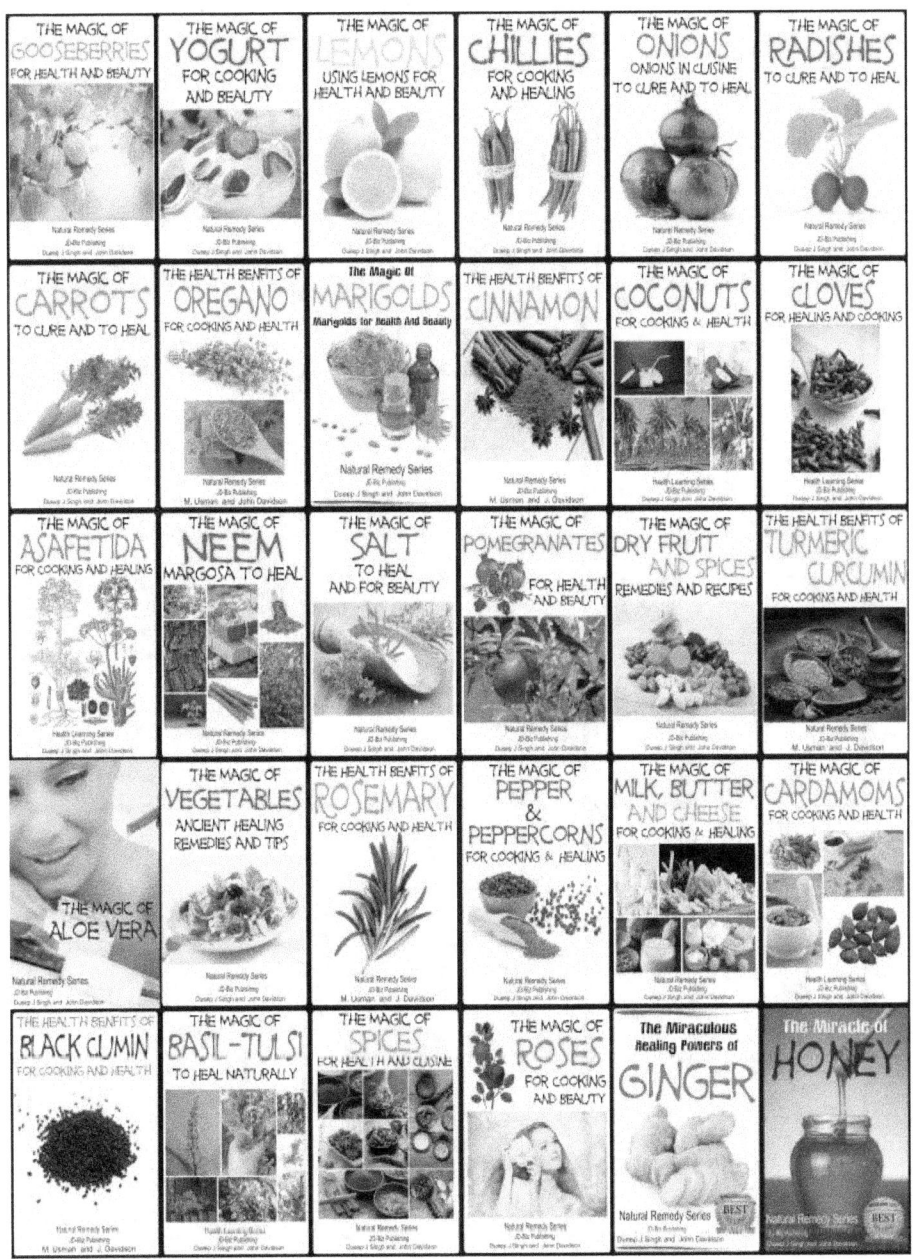

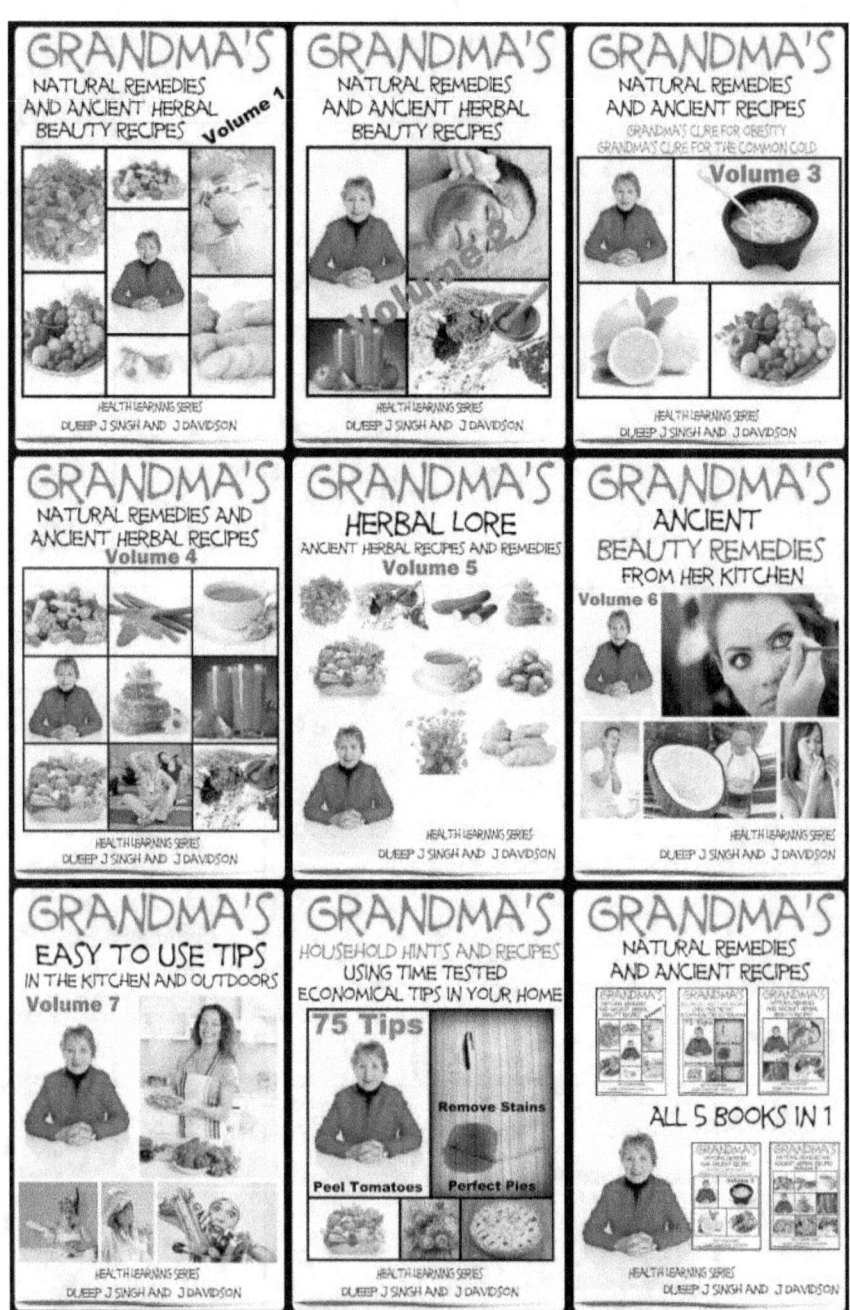

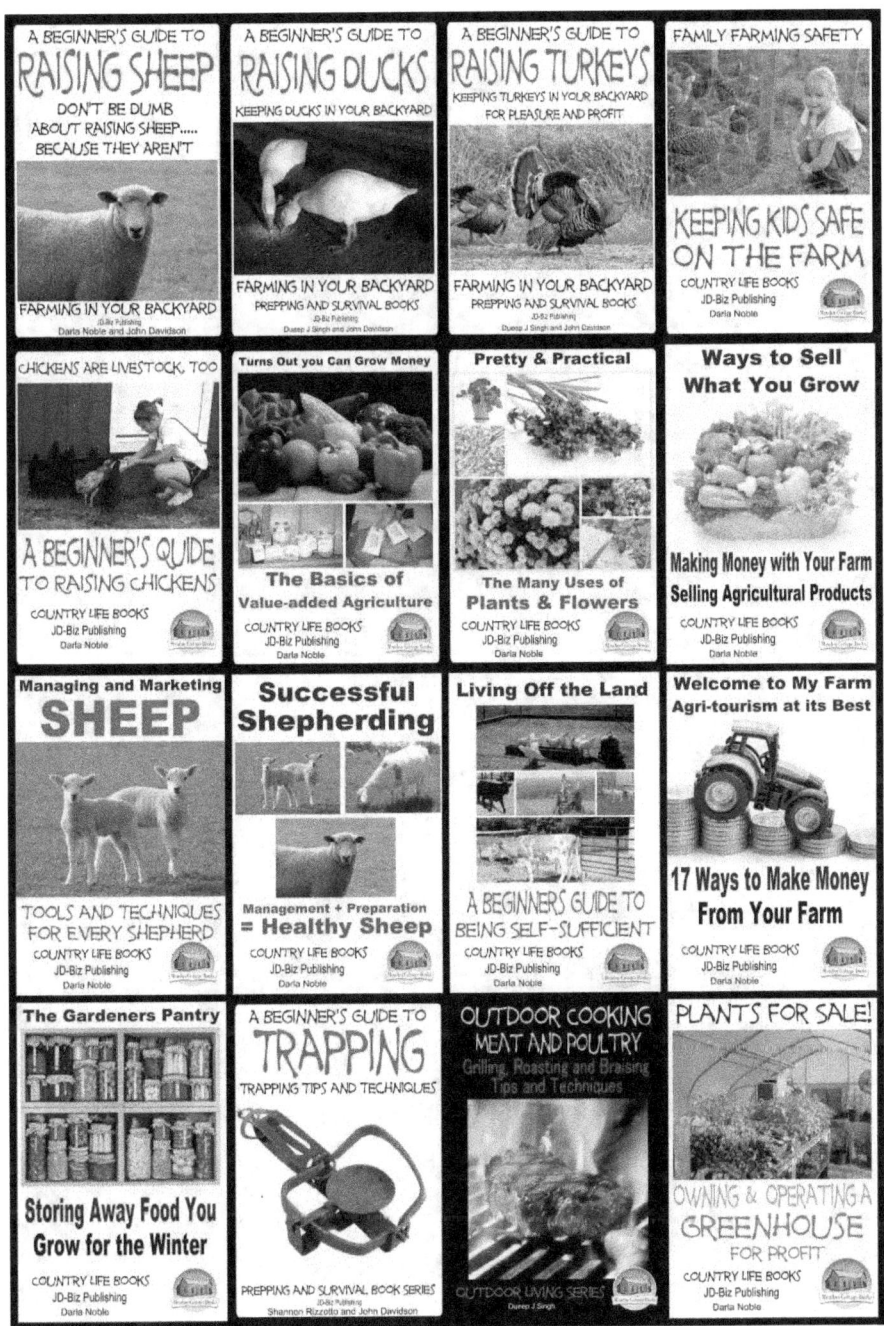

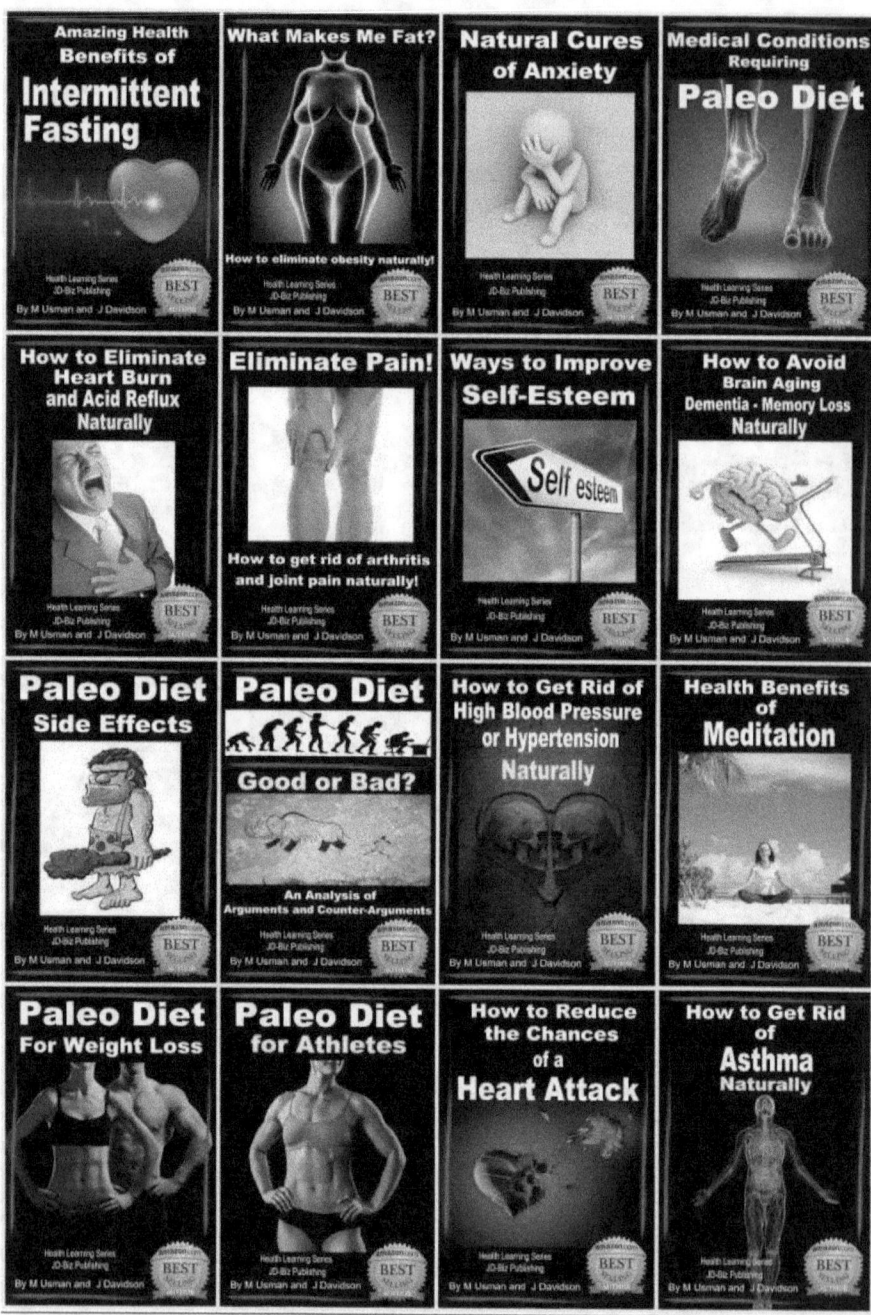

Amazing Animal Book Series

Chinchillas · Beavers · Snakes · Dolphins · Wolves · Walruses

Polar Bears · Turtles · Bees · Frogs · Horses · Monkeys

Dinosaurs · Sharks · Whales · Spiders · Big Cats · Big Mammals of Yellowstone

Animals of Australia · Sasquatch - Yeti Abominable Snowman Bigfoot · Giant Panda Bears · Kittens · Komodo Dragons · Lady Bugs

Animals of North America · Meerkats · Birds of North America · Penguins · Hamsters · Elephants

Learn To Draw Series

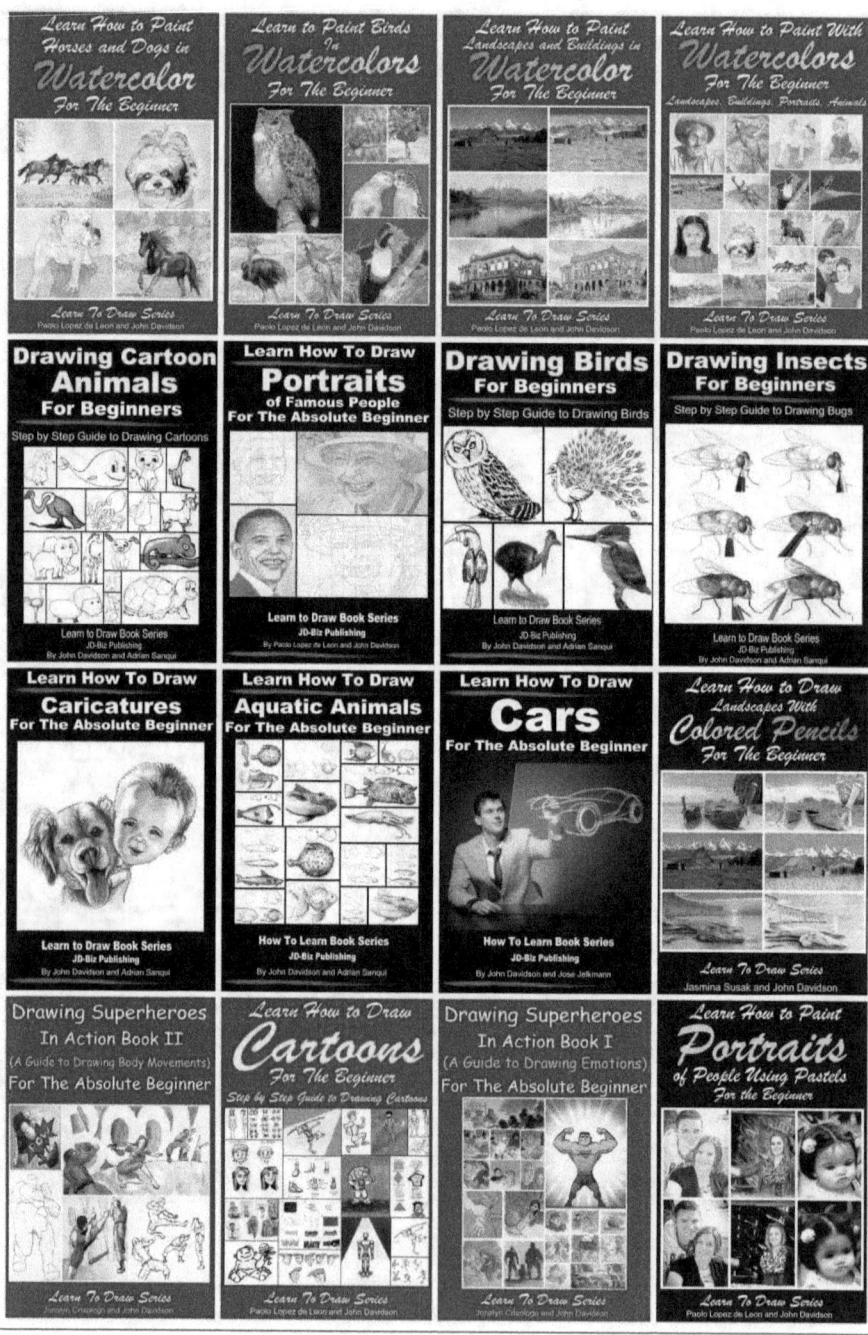

How to Build and Plan Books

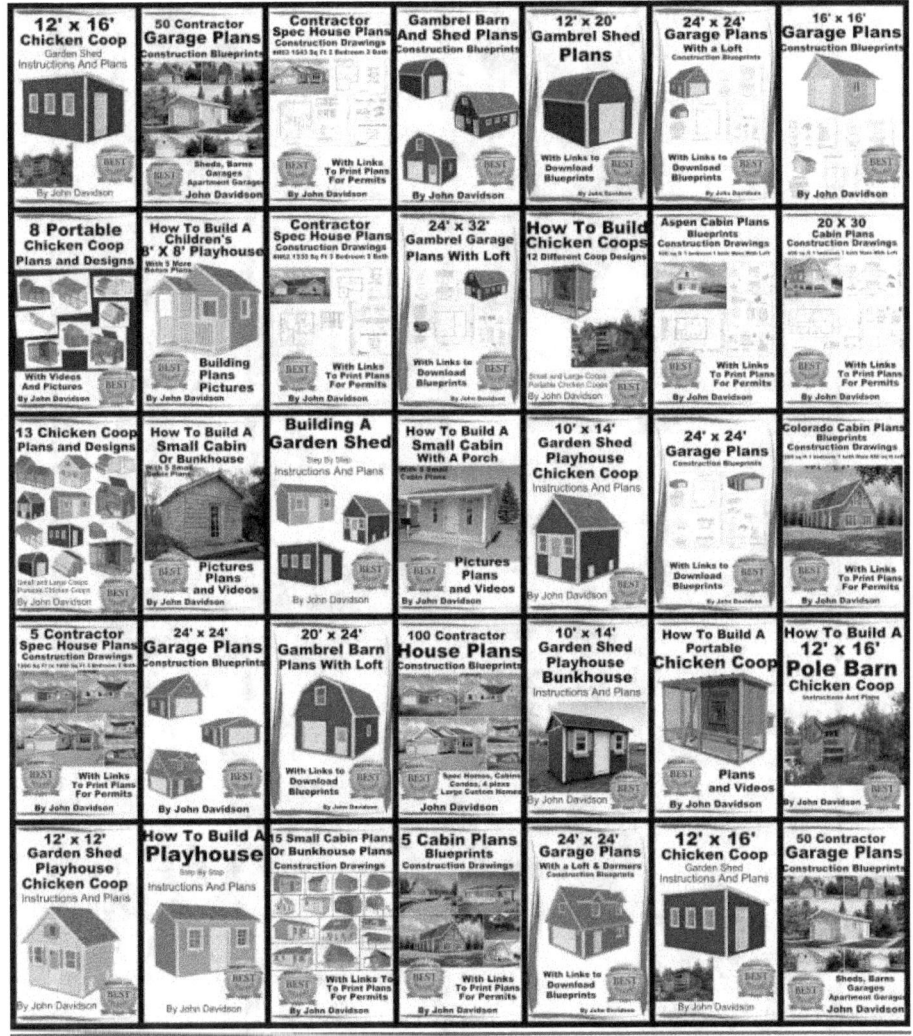

Entrepreneur Book Series

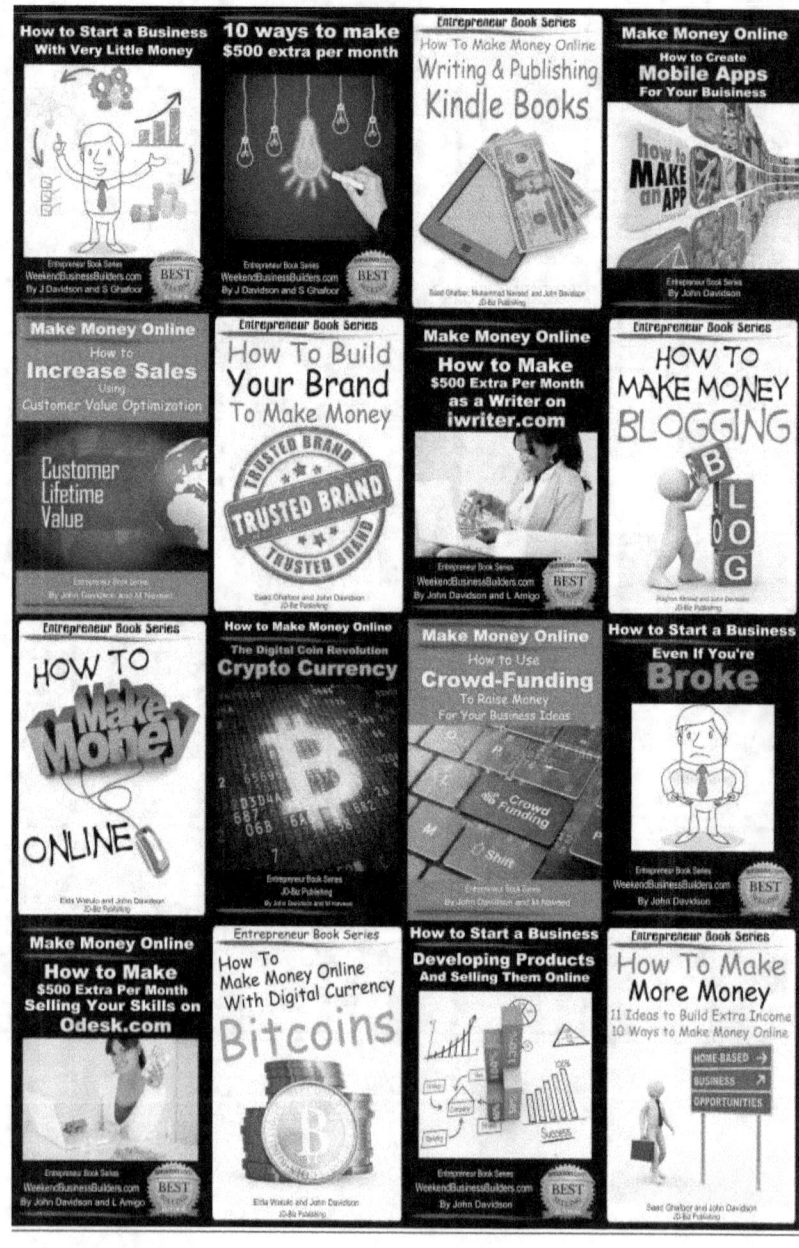

Our books are available at

1. Amazon.com

2. Barnes and Noble

3. Itunes

4. Kobo

5. Smashwords

6. Google Play Books

Publisher

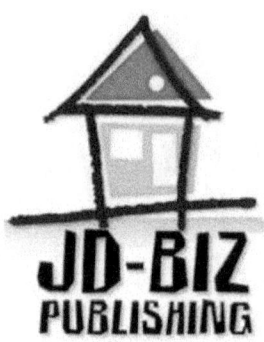

JD-Biz Corp

P O Box 374

Mendon, Utah 84325

http://www.jd-biz.com/

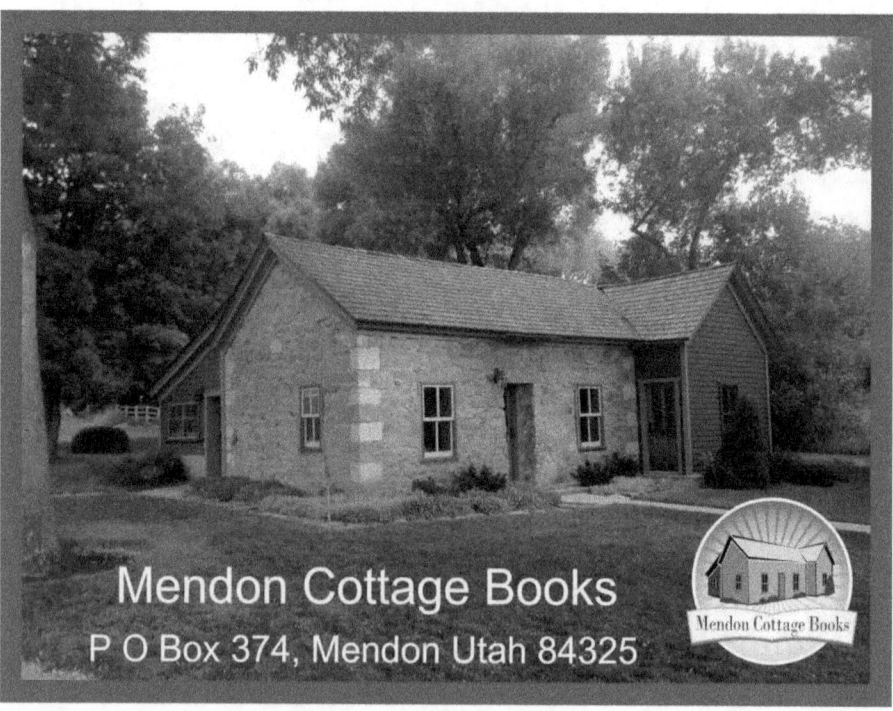

Mendon Cottage Books

P O Box 374, Mendon Utah 84325

www.ingramcontent.com/pod-product-compliance
Lightning Source LLC
Chambersburg PA
CBHW070342290526
45791CB00003B/1438